YOUR KNOWLEDGE HAS VALUE

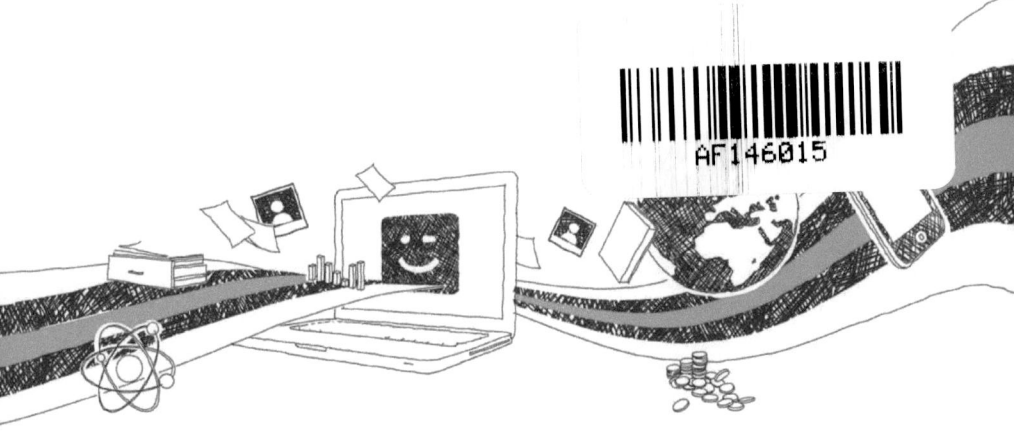

AF146015

- We will publish your bachelor's and
  master's thesis, essays and papers

- Your own eBook and book -
  sold worldwide in all relevant shops

- Earn money with each sale

Upload your text at www.GRIN.com
and publish for free

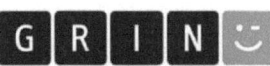

Bibliographic information published by the German National Library:

The German National Library lists this publication in the National Bibliography; detailed bibliographic data are available on the Internet at http://dnb.dnb.de .

Imprint:

Copyright © 2018 GRIN Verlag
Print and binding: Books on Demand GmbH, Norderstedt Germany
ISBN: 9783668702813

This book at GRIN:

https://www.grin.com/document/425372

Sagar Pamu

Adverse Drug Reactions (ADRs)

GRIN Verlag

GRIN - Your knowledge has value

Since its foundation in 1998, GRIN has specialized in publishing academic texts by students, college teachers and other academics as e-book and printed book. The website www.grin.com is an ideal platform for presenting term papers, final papers, scientific essays, dissertations and specialist books.

A Monograph on

Adverse Drug Reactions

Author

Sagar Pamu

List of Contents

INTRODUCTION

DEFINITION [1,2]

The WHO defines an "Adverse Drug Reaction as any response to a drug which is noxious and unintended and which occurs or doses normally used in a man of prophylaxis diagnosis or therapy of disease or for the modification of physiologic function".

Adverse Drug Reactions (ADRs) are types of Adverse Drug Events (ADEs). Adverse Drug Events include ADRs, prescription errors, medication errors and other drug-related problems. ADEs are the negative consequences' of drug misadventures. Henri Manasse defined drug misadventure as the iatrogenic hazard that is an inherent risk when drug therapy is indicated.

The American Society of Health-System Pharmacists (ASHP) defines significant ADRs as an unexpected, unintended, undesired, or excessive response to a drug that includes the following. [3,4,5]

❖ Requires discontinuing the drug

❖ Requires changing the drug therapy

❖ Requires modifying the dose

❖ Necessitates admission to the hospital

❖ Prolongs stay in a healthcare facility

❖ Necessitates supportive treatment

❖ Significantly complicates diagnosis

❖ Negatively affects prognosis or results in temporary or permanent harm, disability or death.

Pharmacovigilance is an integral part of drug therapy. But it is still not widely practised in the hospitals of India. In many studies, adverse drug reactions have been considered as a leading cause of morbidity and mortality. The incidence of adverse drug reactions varies with studies which show incidences ranging from as low as 0.15% to as high as 30%. Older adults and hospitalized in-patients are shown to be more susceptible to ADRs than the adult population (16.6% *vs.* 4.1%). Indian reports on ADR monitoring have been very few. This may be because ADR monitoring is still evolving here. After decades of hibernation, the need for an efficient pharmacovigilance programme was felt, the result of which was the institution of National Pharmacovigilance Programme in November 2004. Under this programme, the Central Drugs Standards Control Organization, New Delhi officiates as the central coordinating body under which two zonal, five regional and 24 peripheral centres have been established. The objective of this programme is to create awareness among the health professionals on ADR monitoring and to encourage a reporting culture. [3]

Hospital-based ADR monitoring and reporting programmes aim to identify and quantify the risks associated with the use of drugs. This is important information which is useful in identifying and minimizing the ADRs where it can be preventable and generally enhances the knowledge of the physicians to deal with ADRs more efficiently and effectively. The participation of pharmacists in national pharmacovigilance programmes is not a common feature. The pharmacist's involvement in such programmes is seen only in some countries. In India, clinical pharmacy is still evolving and hence, pharmacists involvement in such activities has been low. The aim of the present study was to undertake ADR monitoring in a government hospital where a clinical pharmacy programme is well established. The primary objectives included monitoring and documenting ADRs and evaluating them according to set criteria. The secondary objective was to analyze the cost burden involved in managing ADRs.[6]

INCIDENCE[7-10]

The frequency of ADRs in the general population is unknown. However, the reported rates of new occurrences for ADRs are noted for selected patient populations. A meta-analysis of 39 prospective studies reported an overall incidence of serious ADRs in hospitalized patients of 6.7% and of fatal ADRs of 0.32%. The fatality rate makes ADRs the fourth to the sixth leading cause of death in the United States. Another meta-analysis of 36 studies indicated that approximately 5% of hospital admissions are due to ADRs. The costs of ADRs are estimated to be $1.56-$4 billion in direct hospital costs per year in the United States.

CLASSIFICATION OF ADVERSE DRUG REACTIONS [11]

According to the Wills & Brown classification, these ADRs are classified

Type A: Augmented Reactions

Type A reactions are dose-related actions of a medicine upon the human body, which could have been predicted based upon a knowledge of the mode of action and pharmacology of a drug or excipient. These reactions can only occur while the subject is still receiving the preparation and improve partially or completely when the causative agent is withdrawn or the dose reduced.

Type B: Bugs Reactions

These are adverse reactions that rely upon promoting the growth of certain microorganisms. These type B reactions are pharmacologically predictable events, but they do not type A according to the definition used in the preceding section since the direct and principal pharmacological action is on the bodies of microorganism rather than on the human body. Examples include sugar-containing medicines promoting dental caries, antibiotics causing overgrowth of resistant bacterial species in the intestine, broad-spectrum antibiotics causing oral thrush and over the use of one agent stimulating the development of resistance among a specific species of microorganism rendering further use of the agent ineffective.

Note that an infection arising as a result of drug-induced immune-suppression would not be a type B reaction. The primary adverse event in such a case would be suppression of the human immune system, which is usually a type A reaction. Infections arising as a result of this would be a secondary event.

Type C: Chemical Reactions

A number of adverse reactions depend upon the chemical nature of a drug or excipient rather than pharmacological properties. They are all basically forms of chemical irritation, which makes it likely that, when exposed to the preparation, most people could experience a similar reaction. The severity of a type C reaction is more a function of the concentration of the offending substance than dose.

The side-effects which are typical in this category include extravasation reactions, vein inflammation, inflammation and pain at the site of an injection owing to the irritant action of a drug or excipient, acid or alkali burns, contact (irritant) dermatitis and gastrointestinal mucosa damage caused by the local irritant action. All these reactions are not so predictable pharmacologically, but knowledge may enable on the physicochemical characteristics of the causative agents to be foreseen on them.

Type D: Delivery Reactions

A variety of adverse reactions occur as a specific consequence of the method of drug delivery. These reactions do not depend upon the chemical or pharmacological properties of the constituents of the preparation but occur because of the physical nature of the formulation and/or the method of administration. These reactions will be heterogeneous. Methods of delivery vary and so the specific nature of the adverse reactions must also vary.

The unifying characteristic is that, if the method of delivery is changed, the adverse reaction will cease to occur. Examples such as inflammation or fibrosis around implants, thrombosis or occlusion of blood vessel due to injection particles, a tablet lodging in the throat, inhaling the 'dust cap' of an inhaler, cough after using a dry powder inhaler, infections at the site of an injection (owing to the opening of a port of entry for bacteria) and infections because of contamination of injection solution with microorganisms.

Type E: Exit Reactions

These are known as withdrawal reactions and are a manifestation of physical dependence. It is only possible for them to occur after administration of the medicine has ceased or the dose suddenly reduced. Unlike all other adverse reactions, which typically worsen if the causative agent is continued, the reintroduction of the drug will actually ameliorate symptoms. The likelihood of a reaction is linked more to the duration of administration than dose. In addition, although these reactions are pharmacologically predictable to an extent, the development of withdrawal reactions is not universal. Many patients do not experience them despite continuous high dose exposure.

Type F: Familial Reaction

Certain adverse drug reactions occur only in susceptible individuals with genetically determined, inherited metabolic disorders. Some of the more common familial disorders include phenylketonuria, glucose 6-phosphate dehydrogenase deficiency; esterase inhibitor deficiency, porphyria and sickle cell anaemia.

These reactions must not be confused with those that occur because of the normal variation inability to metabolize a drug among the population. For example, up to 10% of the population of the western world are deficient in CYP 2D6. However, this does not make them liable to suffer unique adverse effects compared with the rest of the population.

Type G: Genotoxicity Reactions

A number of drugs can produce genetic damage in humans. Notably, some are potentially carcinogenic or genotoxic. Some, but not all, teratogenic agents damage genetic material within the foetus.

Type H: Hypersensitivity Reactions

These are side-effects caused by allergy or hypersensitivity. They are probably the most common adverse reactions after Type A reactions. There are many different types, but all involve activation of an immune response. They are not pharmacologically predictable and neither are they dose-related according to the definition of 'dose-dependent' given above (although very small doses can sometimes be used for desensitization). Accordingly, reducing the dose does not usually lead to amelioration of symptoms; the drug must be stopped. Some examples are anaphylaxis, allergic skin rashes, Stevens-Johnson syndrome,

photoallergy, acute angioedema, hypersensitivity, cholestasis and hypersensitivity mediated blood dyscrasias.

Type U: Unclassified Reactions

Some ADRs have a mechanism that is not understood and these must remain unclassified until more is known about them. This may necessitate the introduction of new adverse reaction categories in the future. Examples include drug-induced taste disturbance, muscular adverse effects of Simvastatin, and nausea and vomiting after a gaseous general anaesthetic. The severity of the reaction was determined according to Hartwig et al. as given below [12]

Mild reactions which were self-limiting and able to resolve over time without treatment and did not contribute to the prolongation of the length of stay.

Moderate ADRs were defined as those that required therapeutic intervention and hospitalization prolonged by 1 day but resolved in <24 h or change in drug therapy or specific treatment to prevent a further outcome.

Severe ADRs were those that were life-threatening, producing disability and those that prolonged hospital stay or led to hospitalization required intensive medical care or led to the death of the patient.[12,13]

Patient outcomes were reported as:

- Fatal

- Fully recovered (Patient fully recovered during hospitalization)

- Recovering (Patient recovering, but not fully recovered during hospitalization)

- Unknown (not documented)

DRUG HYPERSENSITIVITY

The terms "drug allergy," "drug hypersensitivity" and "drug reaction" are often used interchangeably. Drug reactions encompass all adverse events related to drug administration, regardless of aetiology. Drug hypersensitivity is defined as an immune-mediated response to a drug agent in a sensitized patient. Drug allergy is restricted specifically to a reaction mediated by IgE. Drug reactions can be classified into immunologic and nonimmunologic etiologies. The majority (75 to 80 percent) of adverse drug reactions are caused by predictable, non- immunologic effects. The remaining 20 to 25 percent of adverse drug events are caused by unpredictable effects that may or may not be immune-mediated. Immune-mediated reactions account for 5 to 10 percent of all drug reactions and constitute true drug hypersensitivity, with IgE-mediated drug allergies falling into this category.

IMMUNOLOGIC AND NONIMMUNOLOGIC DRUG REACTIONS[14,15]

TYPE	EXAMPLE
IMMUNOLOGIC	
Type I reaction (IgE-mediated)	Anaphylaxis from β-lactam antibiotic
Type II reaction (cytotoxic)	Hemolytic anaemia from penicillin
Type III reaction (immune complex)	Serum sickness from anti-thymocyte globulin
	Contact dermatitis from topical antihistamine
Type IV reaction (delayed, cell-mediated)	
Specific T-cell activation	Morbilliform rash from sulphonamides
Fas/Fas ligand-induced apoptosis	Stevens-Johnson syndrome
	Toxic epidermal necrolysis
Other	Drug-induced, lupus-like syndrome
	Anticonvulsant hypersensitivity syndrome
NONIMMUNOLOGIC	
Predictable	
Pharmacologic side effect	Dry mouth from antihistamines
A secondary	Thrush while taking antibiotics

TYPE	EXAMPLE
pharmacologic side effect	
Drug toxicity	Hepatotoxicity from Methotrexate
Drug-drug interactions	Seizure from Theophylline while taking Erythromycin
Drug overdose	Seizure from excessive Lidocaine (Xylocaine)
Unpredictable	
Pseudoallergic	Anaphylactoid reaction after radiocontrast media
Idiosyncratic	Hemolytic anaemia in a patient with G6PD deficiency after Primaquine therapy
Intolerance	Tinnitus after a single, small dose of Aspirin

The following classification describes the predominant immune mechanisms that lead to clinical symptoms of drug hypersensitivity. This classification includes: Type I reactions (IgE-mediated); Type II reactions (cytotoxic); Type III reactions (immune complex); and Type IV reactions (delayed, cell-mediated). However, some drug hypersensitivity reactions are difficult to classify because of a lack of evidence supporting a predominant immunologic mechanism. These include certain cutaneous drug reactions (i.e., maculopapular rashes, erythroderma, exfoliative dermatitis, and fixed drug reactions) and specific drug hypersensitivity syndrome.

IMMUNE REACTION, ITS MECHANISM, CLINICAL MANIFESTATIONS AND TIMINGS

IMMUNE REACTION	MECHANISM	CLINICAL MANIFESTATIONS	TIMING OF REACTIONS
Type I (IgE-mediated)	Drug-IgE complex binding to mast cells with release of histamine, inflammatory mediators	Urticaria, angioedema, bronchospasm, pruritus, vomiting, diarrhea, anaphylaxis	Minutes to hours after drug exposure
Type II (cytotoxic)	Specific IgG or IgM antibodies directed at drug-hapten coated cells	Hemolytic anaemia, neutropenia, thrombocytopenia	Variable
Type III (immune complex)	Tissue deposition of drug-antibody complexes with complement activation and inflammation	Serum sickness, fever, rash, arthralgias, lymphadenopathy, urticaria, glomerulonephritis, vasculitis	1 to 3 weeks after drug exposure
Type IV (delayed, cell-mediated)	MHC presentation of drug molecules to T cells with cytokine and inflammatory mediator release	Allergic contact dermatitis, maculopapular drug rash*	2 to 7 days after cutaneous drug exposure

MHC = major histocompatibility complex.

*—Suspected Type IV reaction

HYPERSENSITIVITY SYNDROMES OF SPECIFIC DRUG CAUSED BY NON-IGE IMMUNE MECHANISMS

CAUSATIVE DRUG	SYNDROME
Hydralazine (Apresoline)	Lupus-like syndrome
Procainamide (Pronestyl)	
Carbamazepine (Tegretol)	Anticonvulsant hypersensitivity syndrome
Phenytoin (Dilantin)	
Sulfonamides	Stevens-Johnson syndrome, toxic epidermal necrolysis

Unpredictable, nonimmune drug reactions can be classified as pseudoallergic, idiosyncratic, or intolerance. Pseudoallergic reactions are the result of direct mast cell activation and degranulation by drugs such as Opiates, Vancomycin (Vancocin) and radiocontrast media. From type I hypersensitivity, these reactions may be clinically indistinguishable, but they do not involve in drug-specific IgE. Idiosyncratic reactions are qualitatively aberrant reactions that cannot be explained by the known pharmacologic action of the drug and occur only in a small percent of the population. An example of an idiosyncratic reaction is hemolysis due to the drug in persons with deficiency of glucose-6-phosphate. Drug intolerance is defined as a lower threshold to the normal pharmacologic action of a drug, such as tinnitus after a single average dose of Aspirin.

MECHANISMS [1]

The most common adverse drug reactions are Type A and Type B.

Mechanisms are given in following:

❖ Abnormal pharmacokinetics due to

- genetic factors
- comorbid disease states

❖ Synergistic effects between either

- a drug and a disease
- two drugs

❖ Abnormal pharmacokinetics

❖ Comorbid disease states

❖ Various diseases, especially those that cause renal or hepatic insufficiency, may alter drug metabolism. Resources are available that report changes in a drug's metabolism due to disease states.

EXAMPLES OF ADVERSE EFFECTS ASSOCIATED WITH SPECIFIC MEDICATIONS

Condition	Substance
Abortion, miscarriage or uterine haemorrhage	Misoprostol (Cytotec), a labour-inducing drug (this is a case where the adverse effect has been used legally and illegally for performing

	abortions)
Addiction	Many sedatives and analgesics such as Diazepam, Morphine, etc.
Birth defects	Thalidomide and Accutane
Bleeding of the intestine	Aspirin therapy
Cardiovascular disease	COX-2 inhibitors (i.e. Vioxx)
Deafness and kidney failure	Gentamicin (an antibiotic)
Death, the following sedation	Propofol (Diprivan)
Dementia	Heart bypass surgery
Depression or hepatic injury	Interferon
Diabetes	Atypical Antipsychotic medications (Neuroleptic psychiatric drugs)
Diarrhoea	Orlistat (Xenical)
Erectile dysfunction	Many drugs, such as Antidepressants

Fever	Vaccination (in the past, imperfectly manufactured vaccines, such as BCG and poliomyelitis, have caused the very disease they intended to fight).
Glaucoma	Corticosteroid-based eye drops
Hair loss and anaemia	Chemotherapy against cancer, leuka emia etc.
A headache	Spinal anaesthesia
Hypertension	Ephedrine users, which prompted FDA to remove the status of the dietary supplement of ephedra extracts
Insomnia	Stimulants, Ritalin, Adderall etc.
Lactic acidosis	Stavudine (for anti-HIV therapy) or metformin (for diabetes)
Liver	Paracetamol
Melasma and thrombosis	Estrogen-containing hormonal contraception such as the combined

	oral contraceptive pill
Irreversible Peripheral neuropathy	Fluoroquinolone medications [18][19][20]
Rhabdomyolysis	Statins (anti-cholesterol drugs)
Seizures	Withdrawal from Benzodiazepine
Drowsiness or increase in appetite	Antihistamine use. Some antihistamines are used in sleep aids explicitly because they cause drowsiness.
Stroke or heart attack	Sildenafil (Viagra) when used with Nitroglycerine
Suicide increased the tendency	Fluoxetine and other SSRI antidepressants
Parkinsonism	MPTP a Meperidine related drug considered highly neurotoxic
Tardive dyskinesia	Long-term use of Metoclopramide and many antipsychotic medications
Spontaneous Tendon rupture	Fluoroquinolone drugs even

	occurring as late as 6 months after treatment had been terminated

PREDISPOSING FACTORS [1]

There are many factors that can predispose to the occurrence of adverse drug reactions in a patient. Patients who have one or more of the following predisposing factors are at high risk of developing ADR. The proportion of all patients developing ADR is still very small.

Polypharmacy

Patients with multiple drug therapy are prone to develop an adverse drug reaction either due to alteration or drugs effects through an interaction mechanism or by synergistic effects. The amount of risk associated with multiple drug therapy increases in the direct proportion of the number of drugs administered.

Multiple And Intercurrent Diseases

Patients with multiple diseases are at increased risk of developing an ADR due to multiple drug use for their multiple diseases. Similarly, impaired hepatic patients or renal status patients are also at a high risk of forming an ADR to drugs which are removed by these organs. For example, a patient with decreased renal function who is treated with aminoglycosides is at an increased risk of developing nephrotoxicity unless appropriate dosage adjustment is made.

Age

Elderly and pediatric patients are more vulnerable to develop ADRs. Elderly patients are more susceptible to ADRs due to the physiological (pharmacokinetic and pharmacodynamic) which accompany ageing, and also because they are often taking many drugs for chronic and multiple diseases. Nitrate and ACE inhibitor-induced postural hypotension in an elderly patient is an example of this kind, where the reaction may be exacerbated age-related impaired bar receptor responses to a change in posture. Pediatric patients may develop serious adverse drug reactions to some drugs since all children, especially Neonates; differ in their drug handling capacity compared to adults. An example of such of such serious reaction is the grey baby syndrome with Chloramphenicol.

Drug Characteristics

Some drugs are highly toxic in nature and patients who are treated with these are at an increased risk of ADRs. For example, nausea and vomiting is a common adverse drug reaction seen in patients treated with anticancer drugs. Also, patients who are treated with drugs, which have a narrow therapeutic index such as Digoxin and Gentamicin, are more susceptible to develop ADRs.

Gender

It has been repeated that women are more susceptible to develop an ADR for unknown reasons. Chloramphenicol-induced aplastic anaemia and Phenylbutazone induced agranulocytosis are twice and thrice as common respectively in women patients.

Race And Genetics

It is evident that ADRs are more common in genetically predisposed individual (G-6PD) enzyme are at higher risk of developing hemolysis due to Primaquine than those who are not. Race and genetic polymorphism may account for alteration in the handling of drugs and their end-organ effects.

ADR MONITORING

Case Registries

Case registries first came into vogue as a method of quantitating suspected adverse drug reactions with the discovery that Chloramphenicol could be associated with the development of aplastic anaemia similar technique is of great value where drug commonly causes an otherwise very rare disease which is clearly defined and not subject to diagnostic confusion. The drug must be in reasonably widespread use and the suspect condition must be virtually non-existent in the absence of the drug.

It is surprising that this technique has not been adopted more extensively since these demonstrations of its potential. For some time now there has been a strong argument for mounting a series of case registries for otherwise rare events that are frequently drug related examples of these would include acute renal failure, acute hepatic necrosis, Guillain- Barre syndrome, aplastic anaemia, and agranulocytosis. The advent of computerization should render this a relatively inexpensive exercise with great potential for adding to the public body of knowledge about drug safely interpretation of such registries is understandably complex and difficult if however. Up-to-date information is collected; details including possibly drug concentrations in body fluids will greatly assist the process. Moreover, such information, if rigorously collected, could give an early assessment or the magnitude of any public health problem arising from a newly marketed drug.[16]

Cohort Studies

In the mid-1980s the United Kingdom committee on safety of medicines reviewed its experience of drug-related problems and concluded that, for new drugs used in the treatment of relatively benign conditions in domiciliary practice, some form of surveillance ought to be in continuous operation for the early years following in marketing. In essence, the technique that can most readily address this problem is the cohort study, several such cohort studies have been undertaken and published, a classic example being that in which some consecutive Cimetidine recipients where reviewed over a period of one year during which time all the diagnoses recorded during episodes or hospital contact, whether inpatient or outpatient, were analyzed together with all deaths and the cause of those deaths. Thereafter, the names of patients were noted for further reference by the central registry or deaths and they have now been rollover up over a period or 20 years such a massive exercise has produced useful data on the patterns or adverse reaction experience with everyday use of 12 blockers and has been or value in attempting to review the association between H_2-blockers use and upper gastrointestinal tract tumors. These studies are expensive to operate, however, and the facility to undertake them is not widely available. By 1990, a substantial number of this type or observational over study had been undertaken and in reviewing the outcome, the committee of medicines expressed concern at significant.[17]

Case-Control Studies

Case-control studies are considerable use in a testing hypothesis about the drug-related disease. The technique is a powerful tool for coming rapidly to a conclusion about suspected adverse drug reactions under certain strict. This approach can be of great value in studying possible drug-related events in defined populations, indeed, some investigators have gone so far as to undertake what is called case-control surveillance whereby they investigate a series of information available from case-control studies include the associations between cholelithiasis and oral contraceptives, venous thromboembolism and postmenopausal Estrogen therapy, acute pancreatitis and Thiazide diuretics.

Record-Linkage Studies

Previously individually designed cohort studies and case-control studies were conducted as and where required. The availability, however, of powerful computers has let to record-linkage schemes whereby information regarding outcome of hospitalization and drug exposure within hospitals and latterly, within general practice, is collected and analyzed to give us a powerful tools for conducting etiological research following drug exposure Finney (1965) foresaw the use of such large databases to generate hypotheses about possible adverse drug effects while avoiding the likelihood of bias contained in physicians judgments. At the time, however, the necessary computer power was not available. In an early attempt at analyzing output from a large data resource, skegg and doll (1977) in Oxford reported their ability to identify and increased the prevalence of eye and skin.

Problems in protocol recipients when compared with propranolol recipients. These analyses were conducted following the discovery of the protocol syndrome; they confirmed the potential use of such large data sources for generating significant information on adverse drug effects. As much more information, the possibilities foreseen by Finney in 1965 have become a reality. For most amongst such record- linkage studies are those conducted by the Boston collaborative drug surveillance program within the group health co-operative health maintenance organization in Puget sound (Jick et al, 1984; Porter et al.1982) other a studies have been conducted using different data sources within the USA (Strom et al. 1985) and Canada (guess-et al.1988). Wayne ray and his colleagues in Tennessee (1987-1989) have used Medicaid data to conducted inpatients studies into risk factors for hip fracture. Indicating a positive association with long-term psychotropic drug use and a negative association with long-term thiazide diuretic use.

SPONTANEOUS REPORTING [15,16]

Spontaneous reporting is currently the major backbone for the detection of ADRs. It occurs in one of three ways:

1. Reporting to the FDA as part of clinical trials; Enhanced metabolism of Phenytoin, Decreased Phenytoin absorption, Impaired drug absorption, Potential for toxic effects Decreases anticoagulant response, Disulfiram-like reaction, Hypertensive crisis, Nausea, blurred vision, chest pain, Hyperkalemia, dizziness, fainting.[20]

2. Reporting by practitioners to medical journals; or

3. Patients' self-reporting to either manufacturers or the FDA. Clinical trials in new drug development cannot detect all the possibilities for drug safety. Limitations in Phase 111 clinical trials include a relatively small sample size, short duration of the trial, restricted populations (e.g., geriatrics and paediatrics), uncomplicated patients (e.g., limited disease states), and limited power for adverse drug reaction detection. Thus, the FDA relies heavily on spontaneous reporting of suspected ADRs. Spontaneous reporting is important in the early market history of the drug to determine previously unidentified drug reactions. This has been particularly true in the last few years because of numerous new medications that have entered the market and now carry a black box warning. For example, Rezulin and Trovan are associated with hepatotoxicity and carry black box warnings. Additional advantages of spontaneous reporting systems include the detection of extremely rare ADRs and ability to identify at-risk subgroups. In order to enhance the spontaneous reporting system approach, the FDA developed the Med Watch form.

Reporting[5,16]

ADR reporting is important when new agents with limited clinical experience enter the marketplace. Postmarketing surveillance efforts have helped in the ability to recognize and identify the earlier trends. The need for reporting ADRs should be considered as important as treatment and overall care of the patient. The Food and Drug Administration (FDA) has legal mandatory that pharmaceutical manufacturers should report all ADRs. In instances of death, unexpected, or serious reactions, ADRs must be reported to the FDA within 15 days. In order to streamline and consolidate the process of ADR reporting, the Med watch program was initiated by FDA. This program enables practitioners to use a single telephone number to report events.

ADR information for Med watch may be submitted via: (i). mail form ; (ii) calling 24-hour toll free telephone number (iii) facsimile or (iv) modem. In comparison, ADRs reported by health professional occur on a voluntary basis. The Joint Commission on Accreditation of Healthcare Organizations (JCAHO) requires hospitals to have written procedures for ADR reporting, evaluating, and monitoring. In addition, the JCAHO requires institutions to have a means in which ADRs can be utilized to improve patient care. Typically, the hospital's pharmacy and therapeutics (P and T) committee review monthly summaries of ADRs.[22] The reporting of ADRs occurring in other settings is still unclear. This is the case with ambulatory or community settings. However, the impetus is to devise means in which to capture ADRs in non-traditional arenas.

ADR Screening methods[17]:

The best methodology for screening for ADRs has not been determined. However, several screening methods have been proposed. In particular, the literature has highlighted five screening methods using clinical data. The five include screening for:

1) "Tracer drugs," e.g., Antidotes such as Vitamin K and Diphenhydramine;

2) "Narrow therapeutic range drugs," e.g., follow-up of computer lab values for Warfarin and Digoxin;

3) Change in medications, e.g., documentation of discontinued medications or decreased dose;

4) Diagnosed ADRs documented in the medical record, e.g., chart review or reviewing ICD-9 CM (International Classification of Diseases, Ninth Revision, Clinical Modification) codes;

5) ADR computer report tracking systems. Although each of these ADR screening methods has been described in detail, limited data are available on the productivity of these screens.

PREVENTING ADVERSE DRUG REACTION[23]

ADRs are problematic in that they cause significant morbidity and mortality. Almost 95% of ADRs are Type A (predictable) reactions, and thus with quality improvement measures, ADRs can be avoided and prevented. ADRs may be prevented with the Knowledge of causative factors and with an increase in patient education. Improvements in the documentation of allergic reactions (e.g., via computer tracking), development of tools to enhance compliance, and application of tools to improve prescribing and administration of drugs are other preventative approaches to ADRs. To prevent the ADRs in health care systems, the ASHP, the American Medical Association (AMA), and the American Nurses Association (ANA) generated the following system of recommendations in 1994:

1. Health care systems should establish processes in which prescribers enter medication orders directly into computer systems.

2. Health care systems should evaluate the machine-readable coding (e.g., bar coding) use in their processes of medication use.

3. Health care systems should develop better systems for monitoring and report adverse drug events.

4. Health care systems should utilize the unit dose medication distribution and pharmacy-based intravenous medication admixture systems.

5. Health care systems should assign pharmacists to work in patient care areas in direct collaboration with prescribers and those administering medications.

6. Health care systems should approach seek system solutions and medication errors as system failures in preventing them.

7. Health care systems should ensure that medication orders are routinely reviewed by the pharmacist before first doses and should ensure that prescribers, pharmacists, nurses, and other workers seek resolution whenever there is any question of safety with respect to medication use.

COMMUNICATING[21-23]

Another key aspect surrounding the occurrence of an ADR is communication. It is important to share with all health care practitioners the details surrounding the undesired event. Communication should include a complete history of past and current drug and medical history with particular scrutiny on temporal relationships. Further, more any current or previous treatments for reactions should also be noted. All this information needs to be documented in the patient's medical record and communicated to all involved in the patient's care including the pharmacist, pharmacy, and the patient.

EDUCATING[24-27]

The patient needs to be educated about the circumstances surrounding any ADR suffered. Patients need to be informed, as their role in health care is also important. They should be given knowledge on the type of adverse reaction and to avoid drugs in the future. Depending on the nature and the severity of the reaction, a Medic-Alert bracelet may be helpful. Educating other practitioners in other practice areas or colleagues is also helpful so that everyone can be on a prospective alert. This is particularly important when an event occurs with a new agent or a usual or rare reaction.

DOCUMENTING[28-30]

It is very important to evaluate thoroughly in all aspects in regards to an ADR in order to assign an appropriate probability for occurrence and to avoid inaccuracies in causality assignment. Other aspects important in recording ADRs are documentation of causality, severity, and outcome. Documentation of ADRs must thoroughly represent complete and accurate findings.

References

1. G.Parthasarathi,Karin Nyfort-hansen and Milap. A Text book of Clinical Pharmacy Practice; Essential concepts and skills.2004, P.No.84-100
2. Clinical pharmacy by H.P. Dr. Tipnis and Bajaj Dr. Amrita,2009,P.No.75.
3. Elements of pharmacovigilance; Be vigilant.Be safe;. Raman Sehgal,Dr.Rajat Sethi,Dr Shoba Rani,R.Riremath,P.No.109-123
4. American Society of Health System Pharmacists. Top- Priority Actions for Preventing Adverse Drug Events in Hospitals: "Recommendations of An Ex9. Aziz Z, Siang TC, Badarudin NS. Reporting of adverse drug reactions: predictors of under-reporting in Malaysia. Pharmacoepidemiol Drug Saf. 2006;16:223–8. pert Panel.". Am. J. Health-Syst. Pharm. 1996, 53, 747-751.
5. American Society of Health-System Pharmacists. ASHP Guidelines on Adverse Drug Reaction Monitoring and Reporting. Am. J. Health-Syst. Pharm. 1995, 52, 417-419.
6. Dhikar V, Singh S, Anand KS. Adverse drug reaction monitoring in India. J Ind Acad Clin Med. 2004;5:27–33.
7. Lazarou J, Pomeranz BH, Corey PN. Incidence of advese drug reactions in hospitalized patients: a meta-analysis of prospective studies. JAMA. 1998;279:1200–5.
8. Ramesh M, Pandit J, Parthasarathi G. Adverse drug reactions in a south Indian hospital – their severity and cost involved. Pharmacoepidemiol Drug Saf. 2003;12:687–92.
9. Aziz Z, Siang TC, Badarudin NS. Reporting of adverse drug reactions: predictors of under-reporting in Malaysia. Pharmacoepidemiol Drug Saf. 2006;16:223–8.
10. Van Grootheest K, Olsson S, Couper M, de Jong-van den Berg L. Pharmacists' role in reporting adverse drug reactions in an international perspective. Pharmacoepidemiol Drug Saf. 2004;13:457–64.
11. Wills S, Brown D. A proposed new means of classifying adverse drug reactions to medicines. Pharm J. 1999;262:163–5.
12. Hartwig SC, Siegel J, Schneider PJ. Preventability and severity assessment in reporting adverse drug reactions. Am J Hosp Pharm. 1992;49:2229–32. 9. Murphy BM, Frigo LC. Development, implementation and results of a

successful multidisciplinary adverse drug reactions reporting program in a University teaching hospital. Hosp Pharm. 1993;28:1199–204.

13. Claven DC, Pestornik SL, Evans RS, Lloyd JE, Duke JP. Adverse drug events in hospitalized patients. JAMA. 1997;277:301–6.

14. Prosscr, T.R.; KamysL, P.L. Multidisciplinary AdverseDrug Reaction Surveillance Program. Am. J. Hosp. Pharm. 1990, 47. 1334- 1339.

15. Joint Task Force on Practice Parameters, the American Academy of Allergy, Asthma and Immunology, and the Joint Council of Allergy, Asthma and Immunology. Ann Allergy Asthma Immunol. 1999;83:665–700

16. Johnston, P.E.; Morrow, J.D.; Branch, R. Use of a Database Computer Program to Identify Trends in Reporting Adverse Drug Reactions. Am. J. Hosp. Pharm. 1990, 47, 1321 -1327.

17. Koch, K.E. Use of Standard Screening Procedures to Identify Adverse Drug Reactions. Am. J. Hosp. Pharm. O'Neil, A.C.; Petersen, L.A.; Cook, E.F.; Bates, D.Q.; Lee,T.H.;Bcnnan, T.A. Physician Reporting Compared With Medical-record Review to Identify Adverse Medical Events. Ann. Intern. Med. 1993, /19, 370-376.

18. Green CF, Mottram DR, Rowe P, Brown AM. Setting up a hospital based local adverse drug reaction monitoring scheme. Hosp Pharm. 1997;4:75–8.

19. Suh DC, Woodall BS, Shin SK, Hermes-de-Santis ER. Clinical and economic impact of adverse drug reactions in hospitalised patients. Ann Pharmacother. 2000;34:1373–9.

20. Jose J, Rao PG. Pattern of adverse drug reactions notified by spontaneous reporting in an Indian tertiary care teaching hospital. Pharmacol Res. 2006;54:226–33.

21. Puche Canas E, Luna Jde D. Adverse drug reactions: an update review of the problem in Spain. Rev Clin Esp. 2006;206:336–9.

22. Malhotra S, Jain S, Pandhi P. Drug-related visits to the medical emergency department: a prospective study from India. Int J Clin Pharmacol Ther. 2001;39:12–8.

23. Malhotra S, Karan RS, Pandhi P, Jain S. Drug related medical emergencies in the elderly: role of adverse drug reactions and non-compliance. Postgrad Med J. 2001;77:703–7.

24. Gonzalez Martin G, Caroca CM, Paris E. Adverse drug reactions in hospitalized pediatric patients – a prospective study. Int J Clin Pharmacol Ther. 1998;36:530–3.

25. Classen DC, Pestotnik SL, Evans RS, Burke JP. Computerised surveillance of adverse drug events in hospital patients. JAMA. 1991;266:2847–51.

26. Prosser TR, Kamysz PL. Multidisciplinary adverse drug reaction surveillance programme. Am J Hosp Pharm. 1990;47:1334–9.

27. Bordet R, Gautier S, Le Louet H, Dupuis B, Caron J. Analysis of the direct cost of adverse drug reactions in hospitalised patients. Eur J Clin Pharmacol. 2001;56:935–41.

28. Beijer HJM, de Blaey CJ. Hospitalisations caused by adverse drug reactions: a meta-analysis of observational studies. Pharm World Sci. 2002;24:46–54.

29. Naranjo CA, Busto U, Sellers EM, Sandor P, Ruiz I, Roberts EA, Janecek E, Domecq C, Greenblatt DJ. A method for estimating the probability of adverse drug reactions. Clin Pharmacol Ther. 1981;80:289–95.

30. Jose J, Rao PG. Pattern of adverse drug reactions notified by spontaneous reporting in an Indian tertiary care teaching hospital. Pharmacol Res. 2006;54:226–33.

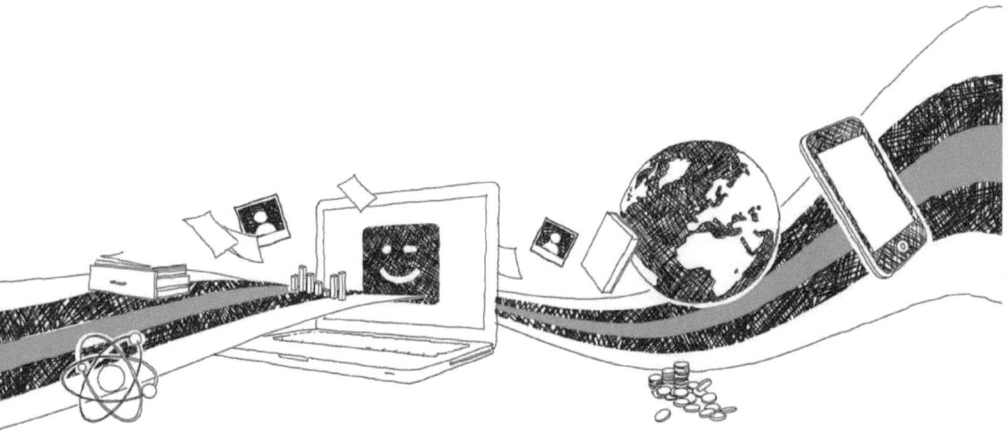
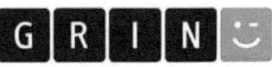